# Gastrointestinal System Nursing Review

A study guide for nursing students to increase retention and PASS nursing exams

Anna Curran, RN

# Introduction

I want to thank you and congratulate you for downloading the book,

*"Gastrointestinal System Nursing Review*."

By

NurseStudy.Net is the Internet's leading resource for nursing students. We offer over **1000 FREE nursing care plans, nursing diagnosis**, and much more. Our Mission is simple: to help nursing students succeed.

We provide the resources you need to succeed in your studies and make a difference in the lives of your patients. Visit NurseStudy.Net today and take your nursing career to the next level!

Thanks again for downloading this book. If you like the book, please leave us feedback and let us know.

# Disclaimer

Every effort has been made to ensure that the information in this guide is correct. The publisher and author do not assume and hereby disclaim any liability to any party for any loss, disruption, or damage caused by errors and omissions, whether such errors or omissions result from accident, negligence, or any other cause.

This book is not intended as a substitute for the medical advice of physicians. The reader should regularly consult with a physician in matters relation to his or her health and particularly with respect to any signs and symptoms that may require diagnosis or medical attention.

# Appendicitis

The appendix is a small appendage that is located at the beginning of the large intestine. Appendicitis is an inflammation of the inner lining of the appendix most often occurring in patients between ages 10 - 30. Appendicitis is thought to start when the appendix becomes blocked by feces, a foreign body, or sometimes even a tumor.

## Complications:

Serious complications can develop from appendicitis:

Perforation of the appendix: This can lead to an abscess (collection of infected pus), or even peritonitis (infection of the entire lining of the abdomen).

Obstruction (less common): the inflammation surrounding the appendix can cause the intestinal wall to stop working, preventing intestinal contents from passing.

## Signs and Symptoms:

Signs and symptoms of appendicitis can include the following:

- Abdominal pain: lower right side of the abdomen.
- Pain that worsens with coughing or even walking
- Sudden pain around the belly button that then starts to radiate to the lower right abdomen.
- Fever: this tends to get worse as appendicitis progresses
- Constipation or even diarrhea
- abdominal bloating

- Loss of appetite
- Nausea and vomiting
- Chills
- Abdominal rigidity

*For nursing exams: tests will usually refer to various signs; however, the diagnosis will be made by lab and radiology studies. The signs you may see on a test are as follows:*

- Rovsing sign: RLQ abdominal pain with palpation of the LLQ
- Obturator sign: RLQ abdominal pain with internal and external rotation of the flexed right hip.
- Psoas sign: RLQ abdominal pain with extension of the right hip or with flexion of the right hip against resistance.
- McBurney's point: McBurney's point is the most tender area of the abdomen of patients in the early stage of appendicitis.

## Diagnostics:

Since the patient signs and symptoms can vary, the healthcare provider may order the following exams:

- History and physical
- Blood tests
- Urine analysis to rule out a kidney stone or UTI
- X-Ray
- CT exam
- Abdominal Ultrasound

## Treatments:

Treatment will include:

- Antibiotics to fight infection
- Drainage of abscess: this usually needs to be done first if an abscess has formed.
- Appendectomy: surgery to remove the appendix.

# Bowel Obstructions

Bowel obstruction means an intestinal obstruction. On the other hand, we can say that in a bowel obstruction, there is a blockage that prevents the necessary body nutrients and waste products from flowing correctly through the gastrointestinal tract. The blockage can happen in the upper portion of the lower portion of the intestine. A tumor or even swelling in the intestine can cause blockages.

## Causes of Bowel obstruction:

Adhesions: Adhesions are a particular area of fibrous connective tissue. This can be thought of as a scar or scar tissue. Adhesions can develop because of injury inside or outside of the intestine or even the pelvic area. Usually, anything that disturbs the tissue in the intestinal tract or almost anywhere in the body can cause adhesions.

There are many different causes of bowel obstructions:

- Paralytic ileus
- Foreign Body
- Hernia
- Colorectal cancer
- Volvulus: twisting of the intestine
- Diverticular disease or Crohn's disease.
- Difficulties in passing stools or impacted stools for severe constipation.
- Intussusception: telescoping of part of the intestine
- Congenital malformation of the bowel
- Swelling/ inflammation
- Tumors: A cancerous tumor can develop into a bowel obstruction; usually, the tumor will cause a smaller obstruction in the beginning.

As time passes, tumors can grow and eventually cause larger obstructions.

**Signs and symptoms of bowel obstruction:**

- Vomiting, and nausea.
- A cramping abdominal pain that comes like a wave frequently after five to ten minutes.
- A bloated belly.
- Having trouble with passing gas.
- Burping
- An abdominal tenderness
- Rapid pulse and increasing breathing at the time of chapter of cramps.
- Diarrhea: liquid stool leaking from the area of partial obstruction.
- A colon tumor is another cause of having a large bowel obstruction.
- Lower abdominal pain; which can be mild or severe. The pain will depend on the causes of bowel obstruction.

**Diagnostics:**

Labs: due to possible electrolyte imbalances

CT of the abdomen

X-ray of the abdomen

Barium enema

Upper GI and Small Bowel Series

**Treatment:**

Treatment is focused on relieving the obstruction and the cause of the obstruction.

NPO

IV Fluids

NG tube to low intermittent suction

Pain medications as ordered by MD (Note some pain medication can cause constipation)

## Surgical Treatments:

A treatment called sigmoidoscopy or colonoscopy. The process starts by inserting a thin, flexible tube that contains a small camera and light attached to one end. The tube is inserted into the rectum and passes through the bowel. A flatus tube (a long rubber tube) is also inserted that will decompress the bowel.

Laparoscopy: This surgery is also known as keyhole surgery. In a laparoscopy surgery, the process starts by inserting a small tube with a light and camera at the end. Laparoscopy may be a helpful surgery for treating a small bowel obstruction or removing adhesions.

Endoscopic stenting: Endoscopic stenting is a treatment process, where a self-expanding stent or pipe is inserted. The pipe helps to keep the passageway open. This process is considered when the patient is elderly or in palliative care of cancer patients.

## Complications:

It is important to note that if the obstruction stops or impedes blood supply to the intestines, infection, or gangrene (death of tissue may result).

Other complications can include:

- Dehydration
- Perforation of the intestinal wall
- Infection
- Jaundice
- Electrolyte imbalances

# Cholecystitis

In one sentence, Cholecystitis means inflammation of the gallbladder. It mainly occurs because of an obstruction of the cystic duct from cholelithiasis. The Cholecystitis is not an ordinary case. It is a very popular cause for hospital admission. Women are suffered more often than men.

**Causes:**

Cholecystitis is mainly caused by gallstones blocking the entrance of the gallbladder. The gallbladder is a small and pear-shaped organ that lies under the liver on the right side of the upper tummy (abdomen). The gallbladder holds a digestive fluid that is called bile. This bile is released into the duodenum (the first part of the gut after the stomach).  In most cases, gallstones block the tube that is leading out of the gallbladder and then causes cholecystitis. It helps the bile to build up and also the gallbladder to inflame for causing cholecystitis.

The other causes include:

- Opisthorchiasis – cholecystitis
- Triosephosphate Isomerase 1 – cholecystitis
- Bacteroides
- Klebsiella
- Impacted stone
- E-coli
- Typhoid fever - cholecystitis
- Secondary infection from gut organisms
- Inspissation of bile
- Hyperlipoproteinemia type 3 – cholecystitis
- Familial hyperlipoproteinemia – cholecystitis
- Sjogren's Syndrome – cholecystitis

- Bile stasis
- Cholelithiasis
- Edwardsiella tar

## Types of Cholecystitis:

There are two types of cholecystitis – chronic or acute, and a rare form called acalculous cholecystitis.

### Acute Cholecystitis:

Acute cholecystitis starts off suddenly. It is a type of acute inflammation of the gallbladder that is caused by gallstones. The obstruction of the gallbladder neck or cystic duct by a gallstone makes an increasing pressure in the gallbladder. The acute cholecystitis mainly depends on the degree of obstruction and the duration of the obstruction.

### Chronic Cholecystitis:

Chronic cholecystitis is a type of chronic inflammation of the gallbladder which has carried on for a long period. It is a pure form of symptomatic gallbladder disease. It makes the walls of the gallbladder thick and hard.

The main causes of chronic cholecystitis are:

1) Gallstones - In the vast majority

2)Cholesterosis - This is called strawberry gallbladder. Here the macrophages in the lamina propria are packed with cholesterol.

3) Ceroid granulomas.

## Acalculous Cholecystitis:

Acalculous cholecystitis is a very rare form of acute cholecystitis. It occurs without gallstones. The acalculous cholecystitis can happen after a major surgery, a long period of fasting, a viral infection, a severe type of illness such as major burns or injuries, and also bodywide sepsis (infections). The immune system deficiency is also another cause of acalculous cholecystitis. Only 5-10% of patients are seen in this case.

Signs and Symptoms:

The main symptom of cholecystitis is serious abdominal pain. This pain usually occurs in the middle or right side of the upper abdomen under the ribs. It may also travel to your right shoulder or back. The other symptoms include:

- Abdominal discomfort
- Pain under the right shoulder blade
- Fever
- Nausea
- Upper right-side abdominal pain
- Biliary colic - spasmodic upper abdominal pain
- Biliary colic after a fatty meal
- Vomiting
- Flatulence
- Jaundice
- Shrinking of gallbladder
- Gallbladder inflammation
- Severe pain in the upper right side of the abdomen
- Back pain
- Itching skin
- Pale stool
- Thickening of gallbladder
- Indigestion

- Yellow skin
- Yellow membranes
- Yellow whites of the eyes

## Complications:

- Infection of the gallbladder. If bile builds up within your gallbladder, then bile can cause cholecystitis. That's why the bile may become infected.
- The death of gallbladder tissue- if you do not treat your cholecystitis, then this can cause the death of gallbladder tissue. As a result, the gallbladder can burst.
- Torn gallbladder- A tear in the gallbladder may result from gallbladder enlargement or infection.

## Diagnosis:

Cholecystitis diagnosis starts when patients describe their symptoms to their doctor. The first one is the physical exam. The doctor will carefully try to feel the right upper abdomen of the patient. He or she will look for tenderness. The next one is the clinical examination. Usually, an ultrasound scan is done to clarify the diagnosis. This is a painless test that creates a picture of the gallbladder. The sound waves of the test help to examine the abdomen. The ultrasound scan can easily detect gallstones, and also whether the wall of the gallbladder is thickened. If there is any doubt about this diagnosis, then other more detailed scans may be done.

**Treatment:**

The essential treatments are:

- Bed rest
- Antibiotics
- Hospitalization
- Pain medications
- Gallstone treatments
- Laparoscopic cholecystectomy
- Surgical gall bladder removal (cholecystectomy)

Medical treatment:

- Bowel rest - clear fluids or nil by mouth and intravenous fluids
- Low-fat diet, once a diet is reintroduced
- Antibiotics
- Pain relief
- Surgical treatment
- Laparoscopic Cholecystectomy
- Open cholecystectomy - When a laparoscopic procedure is technically difficult.
- Percutaneous drainage of the gallbladder - Used in a patient in some cases to tolerate surgery.

# Cirrhosis

Cirrhosis is the result of damage to the liver. Remember that the liver is responsible for taking out harmful substances from the body. When the patient has a liver disease or other liver disorder, this can result in cirrhosis, which is a late stage of fibrosis (scarring) of the liver.

Once cirrhosis has occurred in response to the damage to the liver, it can not be reversed. However, if cirrhosis is caught early and treated, the damage can be limited. But if cirrhosis continues to progress, more scar tissue will form, which will compromise the liver function of removing toxins, etc.

If cirrhosis is allowed to advance, it can become life-threatening.

**Signs and Symptoms:**

Usually, cirrhosis can be asymptomatic (no signs or symptoms) until the damage to the liver is advanced. When this happens, the patient might exhibit:

- Bleeding
- Fatigue
- bruising
- Itchy skin
- Jaundice
- Nausea
- Lower extremity swelling
- Loss of appetite
- Confusion
- Spider type blood vessels on the skin
- Varices
- Ascites

## Causes:

When the liver is injured, it will try to repair itself. This repairing process causes scar tissue to form. As many years of damage from disease or illness occurs, more and more scar tissue is produced, the liver function becomes compromised and worsens. In later stages of cirrhosis, the liver no longer functions well.

The healthcare provider will try to find the underlying cause of cirrhosis to prevent further damage to the liver. Some factors that can contribute to cirrhosis are:

- Hepatitis B and /or Hepatitis C
- Chronic alcohol abuse
- Nonalcoholic fatty liver disease (fat accumulating in the liver).
- Primary sclerosing cholangitis (scarring and hardening of the bile ducts).
- Primary biliary cirrhosis (destruction of the bile ducts).

Other causes of cirrhosis may be inherited. Here are some but not all of these conditions:

- Hemochromatosis (iron buildup in the body)
- Cystic fibrosis
- Biliary atresia (bile ducts that form poorly)

It is important to note that a patient may have more than one cause of cirrhosis.

* Crytogenic cirrhosis is a type of cirrhosis of unknown etiology.

## Complications from Cirrhosis:

The complications that develop from cirrhosis are usually related to blood flow; these include:

- Portal hypertension: High blood pressure in the veins that supply the liver. When blood flow through the liver is compromised, there is increasing pressure in the vein that brings blood from the intestines and spleen to the liver.
- Edema & Ascites: This is fluid accumulation in the legs (edema) and abdomen (ascites) from the portal hypertension. But, edema and ascites can also develop from the liver being so scarred that it can not make enough blood proteins such as albumin.
- Splenomegaly (enlarged spleen)
- Bleeding: Because portal hypertension can divert blood into smaller veins, these veins can become stressed by the additional load causing them to burst.  This can result in serious bleeding. This pressure can also cause veins to enlarge (varices) and become life-threatening, especially if this occurs in the esophagus (esophageal varices) and abdomen (gastric varices). Because the liver is compromised, it is unable to make enough clotting factors, which may result in ongoing bleeding.
- Jaundice: Here, the liver is not able to remove bilirubin (a blood waste product). The skin and whites of the eyes can turn yellow as a result.  The urine may also become darker.
- Malnutrition: The scarring from cirrhosis impedes the body's processing of nutrients; this can lead to weight loss and weakness.
- Infection: Due to the cirrhosis, the patient may have trouble fighting infections. Bacterial peritonitis can result from ascites, which is a serious infection.
- Hepatic Encephalopathy (built-up toxins in the brain): Since the damaged liver is unable to remove toxins from the blood, the toxins can accumulate in the brain and cause mental confusion and difficulty in concentration.
- Fractures: increased risk of fractures due to the loss of bone strength.
- Bile duct stones and Gallstones: this is due to the blockage of bile, which leads to irritation, creation of stones, and infection.
- Increased risk of liver cancer

## Diagnosis:

Laboratory tests:

- LFT – Liver Function Test: This test will determine if there is excess enzymes in the patients' blood.
- Clotting factors: to check bloods ability to clot.
- Kidney Function: Mainly checked for excess in creatinine.
- Imaging tests: CT, MRI, and ultrasound may be done to assess the liver.

## Treatments:

Treatment is aimed at slowing the progression of developing scar tissue in the liver and to the symptoms and complications. Depending on the extent of the damage, hospitalization may be required.

Some of the underlying causes that will need to be addressed/treated include:

- Weight loss: this can help patients diagnosed with nonalcoholic fatty liver disease.
- Alcohol dependency treatment: Patients should not drink alcohol with cirrhosis.
- Medications: may help stop liver damage brought on by Hepatitis (namely B&C). Medications may also help slow down the progression of cirrhosis.
- Ascites and edema: may be managed with a low-sodium diet. If ascites severe enough, the patient may require additional procedures or surgery to remove the fluid and relieve pressure.
- Blood pressure medications: to combat portal hypertension.
- Endoscopy: This is a possibility as esophageal and gastric varices can develop.
- Antibiotics: for any infections that may arise.
- Blood and ultrasound exams: to assess for liver damage and/or signs of liver cancer.

- Medications: to help reduce the amount of toxins that may result in hepatic encephalopathy due to reduced liver function.
- Liver transplant surgery: for advanced cases when the liver no longer functions.

**** Cirrhosis is one of the main reasons for a liver transplant.

# Colon Cancer

*Colon cancer is a type of cancer that develops, especially in the colon. There are many similarities between colon cancer and rectal cancer.*

## Facts about colon cancer:

Colorectal cancer is cancer that arises from the inner wall of the large intestine.

Colorectal cancer is the third cause of cancer in males and fourth in females in the United States.

## Causes:

In many cases, there is no specific cause of colon cancer. Researchers say that malignant cells of colon cancer develops from healthy cells in the colon that have been damaged in some way. When a cell is damaged, it can become cancerous. Cancer cells start to multiply and destroy healthy cells. Cancerous cells can travel to other parts of the body, and this process is called metastasis.

## Signs and symptoms of colon cancer:

- A change in your bowel condition, including diarrhea, constipation and sudden change in the consistency of your stool
- Bleeding at the time of passing stools.
- Abdominal discomfort, such as gas, pain, and cramps.
- A feeling that your stools are still in your bowel.
- Weakness or fatigue
- Sudden weight loss

**Risk factors for colon cancer:**

Some of the risk factors associated with colon cancer include:

- Diabetes
- Obesity
- Smoking
- Alcohol abuse
- Older
- African American
- History of polyps or colorectal cancer
- Inflammatory intestinal diseases
- Familial history
- High fat and low fiber diet
- Sedentary lifestyle

**Diagnostics:**

Depending on the complaints of the patient, the healthcare provider may order:

- Colonoscopy to examine the colon
- CT scans
- Laboratory test

**Staging of Colon Cancer:**

This is done to determine which treatments may be needed to help the patient:

- Stage 1: cancer has grown through the mucosa of the colon but has not spread any further.
- Stage 2: Cancer has now grown into the wall of the colon. There is no lymph node involvement.
- Stage 3: Lymph node involvement is now seen; however, there is no metastasis to other parts of the body.
- Stage 4: Cancer has metastasis to other organs of the body.

**Treatments for Colon Cancer:**

Depending on the extent and type of cancer, the following treatments may be utilized by the healthcare provider:

- Chemotherapy: Chemotherapy uses drugs to destroy cancer cells. Chemotherapy is suggested to give after surgery if the cancer cells have spread to the lymph nodes. By doing this treatment, chemotherapy may help reduce the risk of cancer recurrence.
- Radiation therapy: Radiation therapy uses powerful energy. Such as X-rays. Radiation energy helps to kill cancer cells that may remain after surgery. Your doctors may shrink large tumors before an operation so that they can be removed more easily.
- Medication targeted therapy: Used with chemotherapy in an attempt to target cancerous cells.
- Continuously monitor for complications, which can include perforation, infections, and peritonitis.
- Pain control

# Crohn's Disease

Crohn's Disease is classified as an inflammatory bowel disease (IBD). The inflammation caused by Crohn's disease can cause the patient to have abdominal pain, malnutrition, weight loss, severe diarrhea, and even fatigue. Crohn's can lead to scarring, abscesses, fistulas, and ulcerations. It is also characterized by remissions and exacerbations.

**Signs and symptoms of Crohn's disease:**

- abdominal pain
- diarrhea
- blood and mucus in your stools
- unintended weight loss
- fatigue (extreme tiredness)
- Chronic diarrhea, often bloody and containing mucous
- Fever
- The feeling of a mass or fullness in the abdomen
- Rectal bleeding
- Weight loss

**Causes:**

Smoking: Smoking is the primary cause of having Crohn's disease. Smokers who are suffering from Crohn's disease are at more risk of having severe symptoms than non-smokers.

Previous infection: If you have a previous infection, than it may force an unusual response from the immune system.

The immune system: The inflammation may happen by a problem with the immune system. Immunity helps your body to fight infection and illness. An abnormal immune system causes to attack the healthy bacteria in your body and develops Crohn's disease.

Environmental factors: Crohn's disease is a common issue in western countries such as the UK, and least common or uncommon in isolated parts of the world such as Africa. It proves that the environmental factors (particularly sanitation), has a role in Crohn's disease.

Genetics: Genes that you have got from your parents may increase your risk of developing Crohn's disease, but it will happen if your parents have Crohn's disease.

Age: Crohn's disease can occur at any age, but the chances are higher when you're young. Many researchers' proven that people who have Crohn's disease are diagnosed before they're 30 years old.

## Complications:

Ulcers: A Chronic inflammation can lead to ulcers. Ulcers can develop anywhere in your digestive tract, including your mouth down to the rectum, and even in the genital area.

Bowel obstruction: Crohn's disease can affect the thickness of the intestinal wall. Afterwards, parts of the bowel will become thicker and narrow, and this may impede the flow of digestive contents. You may require surgery to remove the affected portion of your bowel.

Inflammation: Inflammation may develop in the bowel wall. It can lead the patient to have thicker and narrower stenosis.

Colon cancer: If the patient has had Crohn's disease, then it can increase the risk of developing into colon cancer.

Fistula formation: When an ulcer extends through the intestinal wall, this can create a fistula. This causes an abnormal connection between two different body parts. An example would be between the intestine and another abdominal organ.

## Diagnostic tests:

Diagnosis is made by exclusion, meaning that the healthcare provider needed to rule out other possible causes of signs and symptoms:

- Laboratory tests to check for infection, anemias, etc.
- Occult blood – stool to check for the presence of blood in the stool, this can be done at the bedside on most floors.
- Stool cultures
- Colonoscopy/ sigmoidoscopy
- CT Scans
- Endoscopy
- MRI

## Treatments for Crohn's disease:

- Anti-inflammatory drugs – reduce inflammation
- Immune system suppressors – also reduce inflammation but to targeted areas
- Antibiotics
- Bowel rest
- NG tube placement to provide nutrition during bowel rest
- Low residue/Low fiber diet, if not on bowel rest/ Low residue, is designed to lower the size and number of stools.
- Surgery: to remove damaged part of GI tract

# Diverticulitis

In order to understand diverticulitis, we need to know what diverticulum are. Diverticulum (more than one is called diverticula), is the development of some patients as a protrusion or out-pouching of the inner lining of the intestine. They are usually characterized by a small pouch with a thin neck. When diverticula are present, the patient is said to have developed diverticulosis.

Some patients may be born with diverticulum. However, the majority of diverticula will develop or appear at an older age. They will usually appear in the large intestine. Diverticula develop in areas of the colon that are weakened from pressure (hard stools etc.). The out-pouching protrude through the large intestinal wall.

Diverticula can be common in older patients and usually do not cause any issues.

When we see inflammation of the diverticula or that the diverticula become infected usually from the diverticula tearing, the diagnosis of diverticulitis can be made.

The patients that are at the highest risk for developing diverticulitis are:

- Older patients
- Smoking
- Sedentary lifestyle (lack of exercise).
- Obesity
- A diet that is low in fiber and high in animal fat
- Some medications (steroids, opiates, and non-steroidal anti-inflammatory drugs).

**Signs and Symptoms:**

Patients with a history of diverticulosis usually have no signs or symptoms of illness. It is not uncommon for these patients to have bloating or cramping to the lower abdomen. When symptoms do appear, they are severe and have a fairly sudden onset.

- Abdominal tenderness
- Gas
- Bloating
- Fever
- Nausea and or vomiting
- Decreased appetite

## Diagnosis:

The presence of abdominal pain can be caused by several different types of diseases or infections that healthcare professionals will need to do rule out other possibilities.

- Blood tests
- Pregnancy test
- Liver function test
- Stool cultures
- CT scan
- Abdominal ultrasound

## Treatment:

Treatment of diverticulitis is dependent upon the severity of symptoms

- Antibiotics
- Pain medications
- Bed rest
- Bowel rest ( liquid diet for 1-2 days)
- Increase more fiber to diet

## Complications:

- Fistula formation – this is an abnormal connection between another part of the body and the colon.
- Perforation – this is a tear in the colon
- Stricture formation – this is a narrowed area in the colon
- Abscess formation – Area that is filled with pus or infection

# Esophageal Varices

The esophagus is what connects your throat to your stomach. Esophageal varices are enlarged and abnormal veins located in the lower part of the esophagus. This condition is usually seen in patients with liver disease. When normal blood flow to the liver is blocked by scar tissue or even a clot, varices begin to develop.

Blood will start to bypass the larger vessels due to the blockage and start to flow in large amounts to the smaller vessels in the esophagus that are not made to carry such a large volume. As a result, these smaller blood vessels may begin to bleed or rupture, and this can be a medical emergency.

## Causes:

- Chronic alcohol abuse: leads to Cirrhosis
- Cirrhosis: Severe liver scarring. Esophageal varices happen in about 40 percent of people who have cirrhosis.
- Blood clot (thrombosis): A blood clot in the vein that feeds into the portal vein called the splenic vein can cause esophageal varices.
- Budd-Chiari syndrome: It is a rare condition that causes blood clots and can block the veins that carry blood out of your liver.
- A parasitic infection: Schistosomiasis is an uncommon parasitic infection that is found in Caribbean Africa, South America, the Middle East, and Southeast Asia. This parasite can damage the liver, as well as the lungs, intestine, and bladder.

## Risk factors of esophageal varices:

Large varices: the bigger the varices, the more likely they are to bleed.

Portal Hypertension

**Signs and symptoms:**

It is important to note that there may not be any signs or symptoms of esophageal varies until that actually start to bleed. Once this occurs, the following may be seen:

- Vomiting blood
- Bloody, black or tarry stools
- Shock and trauma are seen in severe cases.

The healthcare provider may suspect a possibly of esophageal varices if the patient has liver disease.

**Test and Diagnosis:**

Patients who have a history of liver disease and alcohol abuse should be screened for esophageal varices by their healthcare provider. Some of these diagnostic tests are as follows:

- Endoscopy
- CT scan
- MRI

**Treatments:**

The goal is to prevent bleeding. Once bleeding occurs, the patient can develop hypovolemic shock, and death can ensue.

- Medications to control hypertension
- Alcohol cessation teaching
- Monitor hematocrit and hemoglobin levels
- Blood transfusions if necessary
- Be prepared to give vasoconstriction medications if bleeding starts
- IV fluids
- NPO
- Be prepared to take the patient to endoscopy or surgery.

# Gastritis

Gastritis occurs when the lining of the stomach gets swollen or inflamed. This can occur suddenly, this is called acute gastritis, or if gastritis occurs slowly, it is called chronic gastritis. Chronic gastritis can last from weeks to years.

Once the stomach lining is inflamed, the lining of the stomach weakens and allows gastric acid to cause damage.

## Causes:

There can be many causes of gastritis:

- Helicobacter pylori (H. pylori) – The bacteria enter through contaminated food or water. Once ingested, the bacteria can lead to infection and cause gastric ulcers.
- Alcohol
- Stress
- Use of NSAIDS
- Use of Aspirin
- Chronic vomiting
- Bile reflux
- Autoimmune infections
- Cocaine abuse
- Viral infections
- Ingestion of caustic substances (i.e. poisons).

## Signs and Symptoms:

Some patients may not show signs of gastritis, but when they do, they may exhibit:

- Nausea
- Vomiting – food contents or blood
- Indigestion – burning pain in the upper abdomen, becomes worse with meals.
- Abdominal bloating
- Loss of appetite
- Black tarry stools

## Complications:

If gastritis is not treated, the following complications may result:

- Gastric ulcers
- Gastric bleeding
- Stomach cancer (rare)

## Diagnosis:

The following may be utilized to diagnose gastritis:

- Upper endoscopy
- Test Blood, breath, or stool for H. Pylori
- Barium swallow or upper GI series – these are x-rays to visualize the esophagus all the way down to the small intestine to see if any ulcers are present.

## Treatments and Nursing Considerations:

The following treatments may be used to treat gastritis:

- Antibiotics – to kill the H. pylori bacteria if it is found in the digestive tract.
- Proton pump inhibitors – to reduce stomach acid.

- Histamine H2 antagonists – to reduce the amount of gastric acid that is released into the digestive tract.
- Antacids – to neutralize gastric acid.

Nurses need to educate the patient for the following:

- Avoid alcohol
- Avoid chocolate and caffeine
- Avoid aspirin
- Avoid NSAIDS
- Avoid smoking

# GERD

## Gastroesophageal reflux – GER

Ger occurs when the gastric contents in the stomach back up into the esophagus. It is not uncommon for a person the have GER as it is fairly common. However, when GER occurs more than 2x per week, a diagnosis of Gastroesophageal reflux disease may be made.

## Gastroesophageal reflux disease – GERD

GERD occurs when there is a frequent backflow of gastric contents from the stomach or bile contents from the small intestine back into the esophagus.

Normally, when a patient eats food, the lower esophageal sphincter (LES), located at the bottom of the esophagus relaxes and allows food to travel down to the stomach. This sphincter will then close to keep food products in the stomach for digestion.

But, when the sphincter does not function normally, stomach acid is able to backflow into the esophagus. With the continuous backflow of gastric acid, the lining of the esophagus will become inflamed and irritated. This condition is called esophagitis. As esophagitis continues, the esophageal lining is worn away, causing esophageal narrowing, bleeding, or even a precancerous condition called Barrett's esophagus.

## Signs and Symptoms:

The signs and symptoms of GERD include:

- Heartburn (major symptom): a burning sensation in the chest. This can spread to the throat and even cause a sour taste in the mouth.
- Dysphagia: difficulty swallowing
- Chest pain
- Dyspepsia: indigestion
- Sore throat or hoarseness
- Acid reflux (regurgitation of flood or soar liquid)

- Feeling like something is in the throat
- Dry cough

## Risk Factors:

Certain patients are at risk for GERD. They include those who are/have:

- Obese
- Pregnant
- Smokers
- Dry mouth
- Asthma
- Hiatal hernias (top of the stomach goes up into the diaphragm).
- Connective tissue disorders
- Diabetes
- Delayed gastric emptying

## Complications:

The chronic inflammation of GERD can lead to the following complications:

- Esophageal Stricture: scar tissue is formed from the acid that has backed up into the esophagus. This scar tissue narrows the esophagus and can also cause difficulty in swallowing.
- Esophageal Ulcer: the gastric acid that backs up from the esophagus, can cause an open sore to form in the esophagus. The ulcer that is formed can not only bleed but cause pain and difficulty in swallowing.
- Barrett's Esophagus: this is a precancerous condition in which intestinal tissue replaces tissue that lines the esophagus. This condition may develop into a cancer that is rare called esophageal adenocarcinoma.

## Diagnosis:

Usually, a detailed history will help the physician to diagnose the disease:

- Patient presentation of symptoms
- Endoscopy to visualize esophagus and stomach.
- Ph testing for 24 hours for patients with symptoms of GERD but with normal endoscopy.
- Upper GI series or Barium Swallow

**Treatment and Interventions:**

Patients tend to use over the counter medications in the beginning of GER or GERD to help with the discomfort. If the symptoms do not get better, the physician may order the following:

- Head of bed elevated
- Avoidance of coffee, alcohol, smoking, peppermint, **_chocolate_**, fried fatty foods, and carbonated beverages.
- Proton pump inhibitors and antacids may be prescribed.
- Low fat, high fiber diet and avoid eating 2 hours before bedtime.
- Avoid anticholinergics as they may delay gastric emptying.
- Avoid NSAIDS and other medications that contain acetylsalicylic acid as they can increase the frequency of ulcers and upper GI bleeding.
- Surgery may be needed in extreme cases such as a fundoplication which is wrapping some of the gastric fundus around the sphincter area of the esophagus.

# Hepatitis

The term hepatitis virus is applied for hepatic infection caused by a group of viruses which are known as hepatitis A virus ( HAV ) ; hepatitis B virus ( HBV ) ; hepatitis C virus ( HCV ) ; hepatitis D virus ( HDV ) ; hepatitis E virus ( HEV ) ; and hepatitis G virus ( HGV ) . These viruses have a particular affinity for the liver.

### Hepatitis A Virus:

### Cause:

The **hepatitis A** virus is transmitted through the *fecal-oral route*. When a person ingests any amounts of contaminated fecal matter, then they develop HAV. The hepatitis A virus causes inflammation by infecting liver cells. As a result, the inflammation impairs liver function and develops other signs and symptoms of hepatitis A.

Hepatitis A virus can be transmitted:

- Eating food handled by someone who doesn't wash his or her hands after using the toilet.
- Having close contact with a person who is infected. Even if that person has no signs or symptoms.
- Sexual relationship with someone who has the virus.
- Drinking contaminated water.

**Signs and symptoms:**

HAV occurs mainly in children and young adults. The incubation period is: 10-15 days.

*The typical causes are:*

- Fever
- Anorexia
- Nausea
- Vomiting

*The other causes include:-*

- Clay-colored bowel movements
- Loss of appetite
- Dark urine
- Joint pain

*Complications:*

Hepatitis A does not cause long-term liver damage like other viruses.

But in some rare cases, hepatitis A can cause loss of liver function. This occurs suddenly in older adults or people with chronic liver diseases.

*Diagnosis:*

The diagnosis methods of HAV are:

- Detection of IgM antibody by ELISA.
- Test for abnormal liver function, such as serum ALT and bilirubin.
- Demonstration of HAV particles or specific viral antigens in the feces, bile and blood.

*Treatment:*

There are no treatments for the disease. There is a vaccine available for hepatitis A.

Active immunization- Vaccine containing inactivated HAV is used.

**Hepatitis B Virus:**

Liver disease due to HBV is an enormous global health problem. One third of the world population have been infected with HBV, and 400 million people have chronic infection.

*Cause:*

Hepatitis B is a blood-borne disease. It is transmitted through **blood and blood products, sexual route, and perinatally from mother to newborn**. Causes of transmission:

- Contaminated syringes and needles.
- Semen, which contains small amounts of blood, and saliva that is connected with virus.
- Men or women who have multiple sex partners and do not use a condom.
- Unprotected heterosexual or homosexual intercourse and intravenous drug abuse may cause the HBV.

- People who receive transfusions of blood or blood products.
- People with other sexually transmitted diseases.
- Tattooing with infected needles.
- Infants born to infected mothers.
- Inadvertent needle sticks experienced by healthcare workers.

**Signs and Symptoms:**

The sign and symptoms of HBV are the same as that of hepatitis A. But the symptoms may be more serious, and life-threatening hepatitis can occur. Some of the symptoms are:

- Nausea and vomiting
- Tiredness
- Loss of appetite
- Abdominal pain
- Muscle and joint pain
- Jaundice (yellowish eyes and skin, dark urine and pale-colored feces).

**Complications:**

- Liver failure
- Chronic hepatitis
- Cirrhosis of liver
- Relapsing hepatic failure
- Hepatocellular carcinoma
- Aplastic anemia
- Post hepatitis syndrome
- Papular acrodermatitis
- Connective tissue disease

**Diagnosis:**

Detection of HBV Serology:

Antigen: HBsAg, HBeAg

Antibody: Anti-HBc antibody, Anti-HBs antibody, Anti-HBe antibody.

ELISA methods are used for this serology test.

- PCR for viral DNA.

**Treatment:**

Recombinant Interferon-alpha and pegylated interferon-alpha is used in treating chronic hepatitis B.

**Prevention:**

Prevention involves the use of a vaccine or hepatitis B immune globulin ( HBIG ) or both. Hepatitis B vaccine is HBsAg produced by recombinant DNA in yeast cells. Both vaccine and HBIG should be given at separate sites to an individual having a needle-stick injury from a patient with HbsAg positive blood.

The following individuals should receive the hepatitis B vaccine:

- Adults who are at high risk. E.g., health care workers.
- The household contacts of infected persons.

- Intravenous drug users.
- Individuals on hemodialysis and
- Persons with multiple sexual partners.

## Hepatitis C Virus:

Hepatitis C virus is a member of flavivirus family. Single stranded positive polarity RNA. Hepatitis C Virus has six serotypes. This is a major cause of liver disease worldwide, with approximately 170 million people affected.

## Causes:

- Blood Transmission.
- Contaminated syringes and needles (especially among injection drug users).
- Needlestick injury.
- Sexual transmission.
- From mother to child (Parenteral through placenta, during delivery in birth canal, post-natal).

## Signs and symptoms:

Acute Hepatitis C:

70%–80% of people with acute Hepatitis C do not have any signs and symptoms. Some people may have the following symptoms:

- Fever
- Fatigue
- Dark urine

- Clay-colored bowel movements
- Loss of appetite
- Nausea
- Vomiting
- Abdominal pain
- Joint pain
- Jaundice (yellow color in the skin or eyes)

These symptoms occur within 6–7 weeks after exposure to hepatitis C. But, this can range from 2 weeks to 6 months. Sometimes a person with hepatitis C can spread the virus without showing any symptoms. But many people do not have symptoms, that is why they do not look or feel sick.

## Chronic Hepatitis C:

In the case of chronic Hepatitis C, many people do not have any symptoms. This is why, if a person has been infected for many years, his or her liver may be damaged. In many cases, the symptoms of the disease have not been focused until liver problems have developed.

## Complication:

- Chronic hepatitis
- Cirrhosis of liver
- Fulminant hepatitis ( rare )
- Hepatocellular carcinoma
- Death

## Diagnosis:

## Serological Tests:

Antibody- ( IgM / IgG ) detection by ELISA.

RIBA ( Recombinant immunobolt essay ) - Confirmatory Test

## Nucleic Acid Based Techniques:

PCR ( Polymerase chain reaction ) - detects the presence of viral RNA in serum.

## Treatment:

A combination of alpha interferon and ribavirin is used to treat HBC.

## Hepatitis D Virus:

Hepatitis D virus is a defective virus which is enveloped with an RNA genome. It is a single stranded, negative polarity. HDV has no independent existence. It requires hepatitis B virus for replication and thus causes infection only in the presence of HBV.

## Causes:

It is transmitted via blood, sexually, and perinatally.

## Signs and symptoms:

Hepatitis D virus infection can occur only in a person who is infected with HBV. Coinfection means infected with both HDV and HBV at the same time. Superinfection means previously infected with HBV and at present, infected with HDV. Coinfected cases are more serious. However, when superinfection occurs in chronic HBV cases, the incidence of fulminant hepatitis and liver failure is frequent.

## Diagnosis:

HDVAg ( Delta Antigen ) is detectable in early acute HDV infection. Anti-HDV antibody to delta antigen indicates present or past infection with HDV.

## Treatment:

Alpha interferon can be used to mitigate the effects of chronic hepatitis. No vaccine against HDV, but persons immunized against HBV will not be infected by HDV as HDV can not replicate in the absence of HBV infection.

## Hepatitis E Virus:

Hepatitis E Virus is a non-enveloped, single-stranded RNA virus. It resembles caliciviruses but is unclassified.

## Causes:

- The major cause of enterically transmitted hepatitis is the
- water or food supply
- or contaminated feces.

## Signs and symptoms:

Hepatitis E virus occurs in epidemic form of developing countries. Clinical features resemble that of hepatitis A infection. High mortality rate in pregnant women.

**Treatment:**

There is antiretroviral treatment.

**Prevention:**

- Hand washing before eating and after toilet.
- Sanitary disposal of excreta.
- Purification of community water supplies.

Travelers to high endemic areas are recommended to take the usual elementary food hygiene precautions.

# Pancreatitis

Pancreatitis is defined as inflammation of the pancreas. The pancreas is a large gland behind the stomach and close to the start of the small intestine called the duodenum. The pancreas has two functions:

1. Release the hormones glucagon and insulin into the body via the bloodstream. Glucagan and insulin are utilized for blood glucose metabolism and regulating how the body uses and stores food or nutrients for energy.
2. Secrets digestive enzymes into the small intestine to help the digestion of fat, carbohydrates, and proteins.

Pancreatitis can be acute (sudden) and last for days, or chronic pancreatitis, which does not heal and tends to get worse over time.

Normally during digestion, the pancreas releases inactivated pancreatic enzymes that move through ducts in the pancreas and then travel to the duodenum (small intestine). Once in the small intestine, the enzymes activate and assist with digestion.

Damage to the pancreas occurs when the digestive enzymes that are usually released by the pancreas are activated inside the pancreas instead of the small intestine and begin to attack the pancreas. This attack inside the pancreas irritates the cells and causes inflammation.

When acute pancreatitis occurs over and over again, this damage can lead to chronic pancreatitis from the scar tissue that is formed. Once the pancreas is compromised by repeated damage, digestion problems and diabetes can occur.

## Signs and Symptoms

Depending on the type and severity of the pancreatitis, sign and symptoms will vary.

**Acute Pancreatitis**

- Abdominal pain that worsens after eating
- Upper quadrant abdominal pain with radiation to the back
- Nausea and vomiting
- Tenderness to the abdomen with touch
- Cullen's Sign: bruising around the umbilicus (1-2 days to appear)
- Grey Turner's Sign: Bruising on the flanks (1-2 days to appear)


**Chronic Pancreatitis**

- Weight loss
- Steatorrhea: foul, oily stools
- Upper abdominal pain

## Causes:

Some of the causes of pancreatitis include:

- Gallstones (most common)
- Alcoholism
- Smoking
- Infection
- Abdominal injury
- Pancreatic cancer
- Abdominal surgery
- Some medications
- Cystic fibrosis
- ERCP – Endoscopic retrograde cholangiopancreatography (used to treat gallstones)
- Family history of pancreatitis
- High triglyceride levels

## Complications:

Serious complications from pancreatitis can include:

- Infections: In acute pancreatitis, the pancreas is susceptible to bacteria that can cause infections. Surgery may be needed to remove damaged tissue.
- Pseudocyst: This is debris and fluid that can collect in pockets of the pancreas. If this cyst-like pocket ruptures, infection, and bleeding can result.
- Diabetes: Due to damage of the insulin producing cells.
- Renal failure
- Respiratory problems
- Malnutrition: Due to damage of the digestive enzymes.
- Pancreatic Cancer

## Diagnosis:

The following is a list of some tests used to diagnose pancreatitis:

- Blood work: especially amylase and lipase, which may at least 3x the normal values.
- CT scan: to look for gallstones and inflammation.
- Abdominal Ultrasound: to look for gallstones and inflammation.
- Endoscopic Ultrasound: to visualize any blockages in the bile or pancreatic duct.
- MRI: to visualize any abnormalities in the pancreas, ducts, and gallbladder.

## Treatment:

Initial treatment may include hospitalization to stabilize the condition. Other treatments may include:

- NPO: nothing by mouth to allow the pancreas to rest.
- Pain medications: to control the pain that can be severe.
- IV fluids: to maintain hydration.

To treat the underlying cause of pancreatitis:

- ERCP: to diagnose and repair issues with bile ducts.
- Surgery of pancreas: to remove bad tissue and fluid from the pancreas.
- Cholecystectomy: gallbladder removal may be needed if gallstones are a problem in the onset of pancreatitis.
- Treat alcohol dependence: Since drinking alcohol can cause pancreatitis, sometimes within a few hours after drinking. Abstaining from drinking alcohol is important.

Other treatments include:

- Enzyme supplements: to assist breaking down food into usable nutrients for the body.
- Dietary changes: recommend low-fat, high nutrient meals.

# Peptic Ulcer Disease

The term Peptic ulcer disease is given when the gastric acid in the digestive tract erodes the inner area of the small intestine, pylorus, stomach, or esophagus. These erosions cause open sores and can become extremely painful and can even bleed.

Usually, the mucus lining of the small intestine and stomach can protect against gastric acid. However, if the mucous lining is decreased and the amount of gastric acid is increased, a peptic ulcer can develop in the patient.

Peptic ulcers can encompass:

- Duodenal ulcers: these ulcers occur in the first part of the small intestine.
- Gastric ulcers: these ulcers occur inside the patient's stomach.
- Esophageal ulcers: these occur in the patient's esophagus.

## Causes:

Causes of peptic ulcer disease include:

- Helicobacter pylori bacteria (H. Pylori – most common cause): This bacteria is ingested by contaminated food or water. It is found in 2/3 of the world's population.
- Use of NSAIDS (non-steroidal anti-inflammatory drugs, ibuprofen, even enteric-coated aspirin can still cause ulcers).
- Zollinger-Ellison syndrome (gastrinoma). This is a rare tumor in the stomach that increases acid output.

## Risk Factors:

Those at risk for developing Peptic Ulcer Disease include:

- Age – over 45.
- Gender – more common in women than men.
- Use of corticosteroids and NSAIDS together.
- Long term use of NSAIDS.
- Past history of ulcers.
- Alcohol use in excess
- Smoking
- Radiation treatments

## Signs and Symptoms:

The patient may not exhibit any symptoms of illness; however, when symptoms occur, they can include:

- Pain – the most common symptom, can be gnawing or burning. Sometimes between meals or at night. Pain is usually located mid to upper abdomen.
- Bloating
- Heartburn
- N/V
- Unexplained weight loss.
- Changes in appetite.
- Dark tarry stools (severe symptom).
- Vomiting blood (severe symptom).

## Complications:

If peptic ulcers are left untreated, the following may result:

- Peritonitis – the ulcer can create an opening in the wall of the stomach or small intestine, allowing contents to get into the abdominal cavity causing serious infection.
- Bleeding – this can result in severe blood loss.

- Scarring – The scar from an ulcer will make it more difficult for the stomach to empty. The patient may feel full, vomit, and lose weight.

## Diagnosis:

The following may be utilized to diagnose a peptic ulcer:

- Upper endoscopy
- Test Blood, breath, or stool for H. Pylori
- Barium swallow or upper GI series – these are x-rays to visualize the esophagus all the way down to the small intestine to see if any ulcers are present.

## Treatments and Nursing Considerations:

The following treatments may be used to treat peptic ulcer disease:

- Antibiotics – to kill the H. pylori bacteria if found in the digestive tract.
- Proton pump inhibitors – to reduce stomach acid.
- Histamine H2 blockers – to reduce the amount of gastric acid that is released into the digestive tract.
- Antacids – to neutralize gastric acid.
- Anticholinergics – to reduce gastric motility.
- Prostaglandins – may be prescribed for antisecretory and protective actions.
- Surgery – may be needed if bleeding from the ulcer has not stopped or the ulcer has resulted in a tear.

Nurses need to educate the patient for the following:

- Avoid alcohol
- Avoid chocolate and caffeine
- Avoid aspirin
- Avoid NSAIDS

- Avoid smoking

# Peritonitis

Peritonitis occurs when the membrane that lines the inner wall of the abdomen and supports and covers most of the abdominal organs becomes inflamed. Peritonitis can be caused by a fungal or bacterial infection. It can also be caused by rupture or perforation in the abdomen.

Peritonitis will always require immediate medical intervention primarily to fight infection. If peritonitis is not treated, the patient can develop sepsis.

Patients with a history of peritonitis in the past have an increased risk for getting peritonitis in the future along with patients who have a history of **Cirrhosis**, Crohn's disease, **Diverticulitis,** Appendicitis, Peritoneal dialysis, and **Pancreatitis**.

There are two types of peritonitis:

**Spontaneous Peritonitis**: usually caused by infected fluid that collects in the peritoneal cavity. It is also seen in patients who receive peritoneal dialysis.

**Secondary Peritonitis**: this condition usually occurs when bacteria enter the peritoneal cavity via a perforation in the GI tract. Examples include penetrating abdominal trauma, ruptured appendix, and even perforated ulcers.

** *to remember the difference, Secondary Peritonitis occurs Secondary to another event. An example would be a patient who had appendicitis. Then, as a result of bacteria entering the peritoneal cavity, a secondary peritonitis occurs.*


**Signs and Symptoms:**

The patient may exhibit the following signs and symptoms:

- Fever
- Abdominal pain and swelling
- Decreased urine output
- Nausea and vomiting
- Decreased appetite
- Thirst
- Unable to pass gas or stool

## Diagnostics:

The physician or healthcare practitioner may use the following to diagnose Peritonitis.

- Blood Tests: among the blood tests, a CBC will be drawn to see if there is a high white blood cell (WBC) count, which would be indicative of infection.
- Peritoneal Fluid: the fluid in the peritoneum will be sampled by needle aspiration. This fluid is normally clear as it is sterile. It should look like fluid that comes out of a blister. However, if it is cloudy, this is usually due to the presence of white blood cells that may be indicative of an infection or inflammation. The sample will be sent out to the lab for analysis and culture.
- CT scan will show more detail than an x-ray.
- X-rays
- Ultrasound may be helpful.

## Treatments:

Patients with peritonitis usually need to be hospitalized, and the following treatments may be utilized:

- Surgery – to remove infected tissue and to treat the underlying cause of infection in the first place. The source of the infection must be treated to keep the infection from spreading.

- Antibiotics – To fight infection and to prevent the infection from spreading.
- IV fluids – This will assist in maintaining blood pressure and hydration.
- Supplemental oxygen as needed.
- Pain medications – as needed.

*\*\* If the patient was on peritoneal dialysis, the healthcare provider may order dialysis to be done via a different route until the infection can be brought under control.*

# Ulcerative Colitis

Ulcerative colitis is an illness that is characterized by inflammation in the lining of the colon and rectum, Crohn's disease is a similar condition, and both are a form of inflammatory bowel disease (IBD).

Ulcerative colitis causes chronic ulcers and inflammation in the digestive tract. It affects the inner lining of the colon and rectum. This condition can become debilitating to the patient and even become life-threatening.

There is no cure. However, with treatment and care, the patient can have long remission periods.

## Cause:

While the exact cause of ulcerative colitis is unknown, there are some Ulcer theories:

- Possibly autoimmune disorder
- Genetics may play a factor
- Environmental factors are also thought to be a possible cause.

## Signs and symptoms:

Symptoms may vary among affected people. Studies have proved that about 50 percent of people diagnosed with ulcerative colitis have low-level symptoms:

- malnutrition
- increased abdominal sounds
- diarrhea
- weight loss

- bloody stools
- abdominal pain
- rectal pain
- fever
- joint pain
- joint swelling
- skin ulcers
- mouth sores
- Nausea
- Vomiting

**Diagnosis:**

Diagnosis by exclusion is made after ruling other possible causes out. The following tests may be performed:

- Blood tests include CBC, CRP, and ESR.
- Stool sample
- Colonoscopy
- Endoscopy
- CT Scan
- X-Rays
- Flexible sigmoidoscopy
- Barium Enema

**Complications:**

- thickening of the intestinal wall
- severe dehydration

- inflammation of skin, joints, and eyes
- toxic megacolon (rapidly swelling colon)
- liver disease (rare)
- kidney stones
- intestinal bleeding
- perforation
- sepsis - a blood infection

**Treatments:**

Both medications and surgery that is used to treat ulcerative colitis. , an operation is utilized for those who are suffering from severe inflammation and life-threatening complications. Other treatments can include:

- Anti-inflammatory drugs
- Immune system suppressors
- Anti-diarrheal medications
- Pain medications
- Antibiotics
- Iron
- Proctocolectomy – removing the entire colon and rectum

# Practice Test Questions

25 NCLEX Nursing Questions: Gastrointestinal Disorders

1. A 45-year-old male patient is admitted due to liver failure secondary to long-term alcohol abuse. The physician instructs the nurse to perform a close monitoring of the patient to check for hypotensive episodes. The nurse understands that, in relation to blood pressure, liver failure may cause:

A. Abnormal peripheral vasodilation
B. Hypoalbuminemia
C. Increased renin release
D. Increased capillary permeability

Answer: B. Hypoalbuminemia

Rationale: Liver failure disables the body to maintain normal oncotic pressure, resulting to hypotension or decreased blood pressure levels. The other options do not directly relate to liver failure.

2. A patient comes into the stoma clinic for assessment. The nurse understands that which of the following connotes a well-healed and healthy appearance of the stoma?

    A. Purple-colored or dark
    B. Black and dry
    C. Red and moist
    D. Pale pink and moist

Answer: C. Red and moist

Rationale: A well-healed, healthy stoma should appear pink to red and moist as these are indicators of good blood circulation in the tissues. Dark, purple-colored, or pale colors of the stoma is a sign of impaired blood supply. This can cause necrosis or death of the tissues, which usually happen within the first 5 days post-colostomy.

3. The nurse checks the stool of a patient with a new sigmoid colostomy. The stool is deemed normal if it is:

    A. Watery
    B. Formed
    C. Semisolid
    D. Semiliquid

Answer: B. Formed

Rationale: The sigmoid colon is situated in the bottom part of the large intestine. Therefore, the stool produced in the sigmoid colon is formed or solid. A colostomy installed in this area should also produce formed stool, as compared to other colostomies in different sections of the colon, where the stool might be semisolid or soft.


4. An 18-year-old female patient is now allowed to eat following a colostomy. She tells the nurse that she produces too much flatus which is embarrassing for her. After re-assuring the patient, the nurse recommends eating more:

A. Yogurt
B. Broccoli
C. Cabbage
D. Spinach

Answer: A. Yogurt

Rationale: Yogurt has properties that help reduce the formation of gas. A bland diet which includes yogurt can help prevent too much gas, bloating, and diarrhea. The other options are high in fiber and may stimulate peristalsis even more, resulting in more flatus.

5. During a health teaching on stoma care following a colostomy, the patient asks, "How big should I cut the wafer?" The nurse answers to measure and cut the wafer:

A. About an eighth of an inch (1/8") bigger than the stoma
B. Exactly the size of the stoma
C. About quarter (¼") an inch bigger than the stoma
D. About a sixteenth of an (1/16") bigger than the stoma

Answer: D. About a sixteenth of an (1/16") bigger than the stoma

Rationale: the wafer should be cut about a sixteenth of an (1/16") bigger than the stoma to prevent the impairment of blood circulation to the tissues of the stoma and around it. However, the wafer should not be cut any bigger than this to avoid any leakage.

6. A 49-year-old male client comes in the assessment unit with a chief complaint of abdominal pain. The nurse starts to perform a focused assessment of the abdominal region with which of the following sequence?

A. Palpation, percussion, observation, auscultation

B. Observation, percussion, palpation, auscultation

C. Percussion, palpation, auscultation, observation

D. Observation, auscultation, percussion, palpation

Answer: D. Observation, auscultation, percussion, palpation

Rationale: The patient's abdominal region should be inspected or observed first prior to any other assessment method. The inspection includes the color of the skin (e.g., yellowish discoloration often denotes jaundice), presence of lesions, bruises, wounds, etc. Next, the nurse should auscultate the abdomen for bowel sounds. Percussion and palpation follow and should be done quadrant by quadrant, ideally on a clockwise order.

7. A 52-year patient is admitted due to Type A chronic gastritis. The patient's son asks the nurse, "What does type A mean?" The nurse responds that unlike type B, type A chronic gastritis is able to:

A. Reduce the amount of the gastric secretions
B. Make the stomach walls thinner
C. Facilitate the atrophy and destruction of parietal cells
D. Affect the stomach's antrum only

Answer: C. Facilitate the atrophy and destruction of parietal cells

Rationale: Type A chronic gastritis involves the immune system attacking the stomach cells called the parietal cells. On the other hand, type B chronic gastritis is the more common type where in the bacteria H. pylori thin the stomach walls and cause ulcers.

8. A 29-year-old patient came in with a chief complaint of abdominal discomfort. The physician informs the nurse that the provisional diagnosis is bowel obstruction. The first nursing action for this patient is to:

A. Increase oral fluid intake
B. Commence strict intake and output monitoring
C. Measure the abdominal girth
D. Start daily weight monitoring

Answer: C. Measure the abdominal girth

Rationale: The distention of the abdomen due to bowel obstruction can be quantitatively measured by checking the abdominal girth of the patient and doing this on a daily basis ideally at the same time of the day. The other options can also be done after doing abdominal girth measurements.

9. A 56-year-old male client came in with chief complaint of pain. He is diagnosed with cholelithiasis. The nurse should expect that the pain is found:

A. Pain in the left upper quadrant (LUQ) that is accompanied with difficulty of breathing

B. Pain in the left lower quadrant (LLQ) accompanied with abdominal cramps

C. Pain in the right lower quadrant (RLQ) with rebound tenderness upon palpation

D. Pain in the right upper quadrant (RUQ) that radiates to the shoulder

Answer: D. Pain in the right upper quadrant (RUQ) that radiates to the shoulder

Rationale: Cholelithiasis is a medical condition that involves the formation of gallstones in the gallbladder. The gallbladder is situated in the right upper quadrant. The sharp and constant pain is felt in the RUQ and often radiates to the shoulder.

10. A 60-year-old male patient is diagnosed with pancreatic cancer. The nurse understands that the most important laboratory value to monitor daily for this patient is:

A. Creatine phosphokinase (CPK)
B. Radioimmunoassay (RIA)
C. Serum glucose
D. Carcinoembryonic antigen (CEA)

Answer: C. Serum glucose

Rationale: Hyperinsulinemia secondary to pancreatitis is a common complication of pancreatic cancer due to the excessive secretion of insulin from the tumor, which can affect the islets of Langerhans. Monitoring the serum glucose daily can ensure that the blood sugar levels are kept within target range.

11. A 27-year-old female patient is admitted with hepatitis B. The nurse informs the patient that she will be under which of the following types of isolation?

A. Reverse isolation
B. Strict isolation
C. Enteric isolation
D. Universal precaution

Answer: D. Universal precaution

Rationale: Hepatitis B can be contracted through blood and blood products, as well as needle prick injuries and body secretions. Patients with hepatitis B should be nursed using universal precautions such as wearing appropriate personal protective equipment (PPE) which includes gloves and apron.

12. A 40-year-old male client is about to undergo cholecystectomy. He is concerned about activity after the surgery. Which of the following is a correct response from the nurse?

   A. "Do not move for at least 24 hours."
   B. "Turn from side to side every 2 hours."
   C. "Lie flat on the bed for about 48 hours."
   D. "Sit up straight for most of the day."

Answer: B. "Turn from side to side every 2 hours."

Rationale: After cholecystectomy, the patient needs to improve or maintain good muscle tone, as well as efficient blood circulation and respiratory function. Therefore, the nurse should tell the patient that he will need to turn from side to side at least every 2 hours. This can also help avoid venous stasis.

13. Christine has undergone a colostomy procedure and has recovered well. The nurse is about to perform health teaching on colostomy care prior to her discharge. The nurse tells the patient that initially the stoma:

  A. Should appear dark in color

  B. May have a bluish discoloration

  C. May bleed slightly when touched

  D. Will become more swollen

Answer: C. May bleed slightly when touched

Rationale: The surgical site is still new, so the stoma may slightly bleed when touched during the first few days to a week following surgery. However, the nurse should inform the patient to report any signs of profuse bleeding or infection immediately by calling the colostomy nurse or clinic.

14. A 62-year-old female patient comes into the emergency room with acute upper gastrointestinal hemorrhage. The first nursing actions to be performed should be to:

  A. Treat shock

  B. Treat hypovolemia

  C. Control the bleeding source

D. Insert a nasogastric tube

Answer: B. Treat hypovolemia

Rationale: The patient with acute upper gastrointestinal hemorrhage is at high risk for severe deficient fluid volume or hypovolemia due to blood loss. If left untreated, hypovolemia can result to shock. Therefore, the immediate nursing actions must have a goal to treat hypovolemia. Controlling the bleeding source should be the next goal, but this needs decision-making from the patient or next-of-kin.

15. Peter presents with jaundice, nausea and body malaise. He is diagnosed with hepatitis B. Which of the following is an appropriate nursing intervention in relation to his current condition?

   A. Eat small, frequent meals and have rest periods after
   B. Consume a low-protein diet
   C. Encourage to increase exercise
   D. Affirm that he can choose any food he likes

Answer: A. Eat small, frequent meals and have rest periods after

Rationale: The patient has fatigue due to body malaise or general weakness as well as nausea. Therefore, he should aim for small but frequent meals to avoid nausea and have rest periods after eating to avoid expending too much energy.

16. A 54-year-old male patient is schedule for colostomy following colorectal surgery for a malignant tumor. He tells the nurse that he feels really anxious about the colostomy. The nurse appropriately responds by:

    A. Showing pictures of colostomies
    B. Referring the patient to a colostomy specialist nurse
    C. Using open-ended questions to assess the patient's knowledge about colostomies
    D. Give written information about colostomies

Answer: C. Using open-ended questions to assess the patient's knowledge about colostomies

Rationale: Using open-ended questions to assess the patient's knowledge about colostomies can help relieve anxiety. All the other options can also help in the care of this patient and should be considered as next steps in his nursing care.

17. A 49-year-old male client is being prepared for bowel surgery. To reduce the number of intestinal bacteria, the physician prescribes an antibiotic. The nurse understands that the synthesis of _____ can lead to low prothrombin levels in relation to antibiotic therapy?

A. Vitamin K

B. Vitamin C

C. Vitamin A

D. Vitamin E

Answer: A. Vitamin K

Rationale: In this scenario, antibiotic therapy is aimed at reducing the intestinal bacteria for bowel surgery. Antibiotics can reduce the intestinal bacteria that synthesize vitamins K, B12, and other nutritional substances.

18. A male client is about to undergo colonoscopy. During preparation, the nurse explains that during the procedure the patient should initially assume which of the following positions?

A. Prone position with elevated upper body

B. Left-side lying position while bending the knees

C. Supine with straight legs

D. Right-side lying position with straight legs

Answer: B. Left-side lying position while bending the knees

Rationale: The initial position during colonoscopy is left-side lying position while bending the knees. This can help stabilize the position of the patient and enable the endoscopist to navigate the areas properly.

19. A nurse is creating her nursing care plan with a nursing diagnosis of fluid volume deficit. The nurse understands that which of the following conditions is applicable for this diagnosis?

    A. Appendicitis
    B. Gastric ulcer
    C. Pancreatitis
    D. Cholecystitis

Answer: C. Pancreatitis

Rationale: In acute pancreatitis, the patient experiences fluid shifts, which can cause hypovolemia and corresponds to the nursing diagnosis of Fluid Volume Deficit (FVE). If left untreated, the patient is at high risk for hypovolemic shock.

20. A 52-year-old client is rushed to the emergency room with upper gastrointestinal bleeding. Which of the following diagnostic tests is expected to be done first?

A. Upper GI series

B. Hemoglobin (Hb) levels and hematocrit (HCT)

C. Arterial blood gases (ABGs)

D. Endoscopy

Answer: D. Endoscopy

Rationale: the most effective way to directly evaluate the upper gastrointestinal tract is to perform endoscopy. About 90% of bleeding lesions can be detected using this diagnostic procedure. Upper GI series can be performed but has a lower accuracy rate than endoscopy.

21. Mr. Smith has undergone liver transplant. He is now on his 4th day of post-operative monitoring in the surgical unit. Which of the following nursing diagnoses takes primary focus for this patient?

A. Risk for Rejection

B. Excess Fluid Volume

C. Impaired Skin Integrity

D. Decreased Cardiac Output

Answer: A. Risk for Rejection

Rationale: There is always a chance of rejection on transplant patients. In liver transplant patients, the risk for rejection is high during the 4th to 10th day after the surgery.

22. A 70-year-old female client has been transferred to the surgical ward following a colon resection surgery. During rounds, the nurse notices that wound dehiscence is evident. Which of the following actions should the nurse do first?

   A. Inform the physician
   B. Get a sterile bandage and wrap around the wound
   C. Soak sterile dressings on saline and carefully place on the wound
   D. Attempt to close the dehiscence by pulling the edges together.

Answer: C. Soak sterile dressings on saline and carefully place on the wound

Rationale: The first nursing action in this scenario is to soak sterile dressings on saline and carefully place on the wound to prevent the drying of the tissues and avoid infection. After this, the nurse should immediately call the physician.

23. Ms. Stone has undergone ileostomy due to inflammatory bowel disease (IBD). The nurse performing the health teaching prior to discharge should tell Ms. Stone to:

A. Consume medications that are enteric coated.

B. Eat a high fiber and low protein diet.

C. Wear an appliance pouch only at daytime.

D. Increase oral fluid intake.

Answer: D. Increase oral fluid intake.

Rationale: The patient with ileostomy drains liquid waste, therefore, she is at risk for dehydration. The nurse should encourage her to improve her oral fluid intake. The appliance pouch should be worn all the time. The patient should consume low fiber diet to avoid irritating the intestines. Enteric-coated medications should be avoided as the body cannot absorb these following an ileostomy.

24. Mr. Milano has been diagnosed with esophageal varices. Which of the following assessment findings is evidence of this diagnosis?

A. Increased blood pressure

B. Decreased urinary output

C. Increased heart rate

D. Decreased respiratory rate

Answer: C. Increased heart rate

Rationale: The right side of the heart compensates in retrograde flow in patients with esophageal varices. This results in increased heart rate or tachycardia.

25. A 56-year-old patient comes into the emergency room with gastrointestinal bleeding due to esophageal varices. He requires Sengstaken-Blakemore intubation. The nurse should monitor the patient for which of the following complications of this procedure?

    A. Pulmonary embolization
    B. Pulmonary obstruction
    C. Cor pulmonale
    D. Pericardiectomy syndrome

Answer: B. Pulmonary obstruction

Rationale: During Sengstaken-Blakemore intubation, the nurse should check for pulmonary obstruction. This can be a result of the deflation of the balloon or its rupture, which can obstruct the airways.

# Looking to ace your Gastrointestinal Nursing Exam?

Our <u>Gastrointestinal Disorders Nursing Test Review: Master Nursing School and the NCLEX</u> Exam book comes with 125 practice test questions with rationales, so you can study at your own pace and be fully prepared come exam day.

Nursing school and the NCLEX can be tough, but our Gastrointestinal Disorders Nursing Test Review can help make things easier. This test review features 125 practice questions with detailed rationales to help you learn and understand the material.

Don't go into your nursing exams unprepared- our <u>Gastrointestinal Disorders Nursing Test Review</u> can help you ace the test and reach your goals.

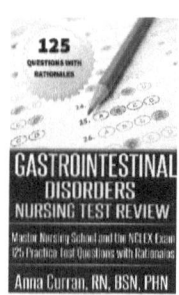

# Disclaimer

Nursing and medicine are continuously changing and evolving. All the information in this publication has been reviewed for accuracy. The information in this publication is believed to be reliable and accurate. However, despite all efforts and continual changes in best practices, the publisher and author, and any other party involved in the production of this information disclaim all responsibility from any mistakes and errors contained within the work and from the results of the use of this information. Readers are encouraged to check all information and institutional policies for up-to-date guidelines.

NCLEX®, NCLEX®-RN®, and NCLEX®-PN® are registered trademarks of the National Council of State Boards of Nursing, Inc. They hold no affiliation with this book or related products.